DEDICATION

This Book is dedicated to my dearest
Mother, who is the source of my
Inspiration...

10 BEST HABITS TO CHANGE YOUR LIFE

A STEP FORWARD TO BE A SUCCESSFUL HUMAN BEING

PRAMOD DHUMALE

CONTENTS

1. BRAIN FOOD

The human brain is one of the important organs of our body. It is also called a CPU of the human body. As we need nutritious food for a healthy body, in the same manner, we need healthy thoughts for the best life. Our daily thoughts create a kind of impact on us. Hence, for the best results always read good books, listen to optimistic thoughts and creative ideas of great personalities, even listening melodious music makes our brain creative. Try to solve puzzles, play brain games; it will help you to sharpen your memory. Scientific research says that if we repeat the same thing in 47 hours then it will become long-lasting as a part of our memory.

The active brain always creates unique ideas and for that, the process of thinking should go on properly. Yoga and meditation are one of the sources to keep our brain active. This habit of meditation improves our decision making which leads the path of glory.

Subsequently, our environment in which we live also affects us. It may give us strength or lead towards misery. The positive environment around us is a source of energy. One can feel liveliness in trees, plants and flowers around us. Healthy surrounding boosts our spirit hence, try to spend as much time as possible in a good and positive environment.

Similarly, nutritionists advise that food like green and leafy vegetables like spinach, broccoli, collards etc. retain our brain healthy. So, eat healthy food, read good books, think optimistic, and stay healthy.

2. LEARN ONE NEW THING IN A DAY

Learning is a lifelong process. You cannot say that I know everything. That is the reason we try to learn all time and this the secret of progress. For that, you need to develop a habit to learn a new thing in a day and of course, this is not a big deal. Once you start doing it regularly you will be habitual and the quality of eagerness will be developed within you. Let us take an example, suppose you want to learn a new language and for learning it you should have enough vocabulary to express yourself in that particular language. In this case, you may start learning one new word in a day and start practising it. In this manner, in a month you will learn 30 new words and in a year three 365 words. Don't you think that is amazing?

Like this, you may do several activities based on your won interest. That is the reason it is rightly said that slow and steady wins the race. But this is just for the beginning to develop your habit. Once, it becomes a part of your daily activity then you have to start increasing it. Instead of one, you should try to learn two or three new things in a day. This is the way you have to continue it based upon your capability.

Don't try to limit yourself. The human brain can do several magical things, you just need to recognise the power of it. There are so many examples of the power of the human brain in the world just have a look of your surroundings.

3. PHYSICAL AND MENTAL EXERCISE OF EVERY DAY

Being mentally strong is as good as being healthy. Physical exercise keeps us strong, fit and fine. In the same way, mental exercise keeps us calm and quiet. This makes us capable to take a right decision. We do give lots of excuses for not taking care of it. Usually, everyone is busy in our day to day lives but it is as important as our daily food to live our life.

For physical exercise, you may go for a morning walk or may join any gymnasium. In case you do not have enough time, Yoga is the best exercise for you. From *Suryanamaskar* to various *Pranayama* and *Asanas* will keep you healthy. It builds your immunity as well as boosts your stamina to keep you healthy.

Correspondingly, for mental health one should practice meditation regularly. It keeps focused and also improves the power of concentration. It reduces stress and blood pressure as well as it helps to lower one's cholesterol level. It improves work proficiency. It gives better sleep and keeps the level of one's happiness very high.

4. STAY CONNECTED WITH POSITIVE PEOPLE

People with positivity play the most important role in life. They are like the fragrance of the flower. Wherever they go they inspire and motivate all. Staying connected with such people keeps us motivated. It is said that one great friend is as good as a hundred books. Both give us confidence, experience, inspiration as well as guidance to move forward in life. They are the torchbearers who show us the right way in life.

Accompany of such people will keep away from the immoral things in life. Try to share your views or ideas with them as well as do consult with them whenever you need any advice or guidance from them. We learn by imitating others so try to follow the people of morality. The same person may have few decadences. Such things are not in our control. It's up-on what to select or what to neglect. Hence, try to avoid such things and follow the good habits of them.

There are so many people around us, we only need to observe them and their goodness. This aspect of looking others will change your life. So, go on, your search starts here.

5. JUST NOT BATHE BUT CLEAN YOUR MIND TOO

Every day we bathe to clear our body but what about our mind? Day after day, months after months, we try to store so much information in our mind. It may be golden memories, happy thoughts, our achievements, success stories, new milestones, plans, ideas and sometimes unwanted or unnecessary things like hate for someone, fights, immoral experiences and so on. Like dustbin, every day we just fill it but forget to clean it. Do we keep garbage in the dustbin for a long time? Of course, not at all. Then why do we keep such unnecessary thoughts in our mind? It's time to clean your mind too. Yes, like daily activity we need to clean it.

There are so many activities to clean our mind but one of the best methods is to forgive those who hurt you. So, just before you sleep, sit straight, calm and in a relaxed position; close your eyes and try to remember the things of the day. If, there is any bad experience then try to learn a lesson from it so that in future you won't commit the same mistake. We cannot control all things but the one thing we can control i.e. let us not allow any incident to overpower our peace and emotions.

So, start it from today itself. You will feel relaxed and as fresh as bloomed flowers.

6. AIM HIGH

Having an aim in life shows that you are just not alive but also passionate about your life and determine to achieve your goal. Most of the people complete their education but still, they have confusion about their aim in life or maybe they didn't think about it. If the same thing is happening with you then worry not. It happens! There is never late until you begin. The moment you start thinking about it your life will change. Slow and steadily wins the race.

As we know that there are two types of Aims. The first one is a Long-Term Goal and the second one is a Short-Term Goal. Long-Term Goal is about your final destination and Short-Term Goal is about your daily efforts to achieve your ultimate Long-Term Goal.

Short-Term Goal is something one wants to achieve in near future. One may want to achieve it in a day, in a week, in a month or even in a year. Your final goal or Long-Term Goal depends upon it. So, performing it in the best manner is key to your success. It is very simple to perform it; first prepare a plan or time table and follow it accordingly. It seems very simple. But don't worry! Practice makes man and woman perfect. So, just go on. You can so it.

Long-Term Goal is also important in your life and it depends upon your Short-Term Goal. Hence, it very easy to achieve but for that, you have to concentrate upon your Short-Term Goal. And for that same things are there i.e. follow your timetable and try to give your best. Be focused and at least once try to remember it in a day. This will keep you focused and motivated.

7. HAVING HIGH SELF-ESTEEM

Having high self-esteem is the key to self-confidence. Sometimes when we self-observe the graph of our progress, we try to compare ourself with others, which leads us towards a kind of guilt and this is the reason of wrong decision making. This is the time you need to learn that there is no one perfect on this earth. If someone is good at one thing does not mean that he or she is also better at all other things too.

There is no absolute comparison between the sun and the moon. The Sun shines and gives energy to all animals and vegetation; apart from this, the moon gives coolness in the night and is a source of delight. In this way, there is no comparison between these two. If we compare apple with orange then is it worthwhile? Of course, not! As apple is a rich source of iron, orange is a rich source of Vitamin C, as well as the taste of both fruits are unique one.

Thus, in our life too, we all are unique one. We all have our special qualities and skills. Hence, all are different and unique one. In this manner, whenever we look ourself in the mirror, we should look with pride and a respectful manner. And talk to oneself that I am unique, I am powerful, I am blessed, I am confident, I am courageous, I am the happiest person in the world, I am creative, I am fortunate, I am talented, I am genius, I am the best, everyone loves me, everyone respects me, everyone is helpful and co-operative to me. These positive statements will lead you to feel very special and confident one.

8. THE POWER OF DECISION MAKING

Right Decision at right time may change your life. Decision making is very important in life. Most people try to copy others but don't you think that you need to take decision-based upon your need and priority. Apart from our main aim, we also need to do various things in life. And for performing it better try to set your priority according to your requirement. It not only will save your time but also will lead you to move forward in your life successfully.

After setting priorities once you take the right decision then you need to be firm on it. It should not happen that suddenly you want to modify it. Of course, without doubt, you may modify it, if necessary but just not make it hastily. First, stay clam think that why do I want to change it. What are the other ways to achieve my goal? And how it will change my life? This is the way you have to decide.

First, start deciding with minor things then you have to take major decisions. When you start with minor things, achieving these minor goals will boost your confidence up. This is the key to success because most decisions are the one which leads to life. The way you are right now is because of your own decisions in the past. So, be habitual to make correct decisions and you will realise the magical power of decision   making.

9. THINK BIGGER DO BETTER

You are the creator of your destiny and you are the product of your thoughts in the past. We always try to postpone our plans and ideas. As per a scientific survey, it is proved that most of the humans live in their dreams, sometimes of past and frequently about their future and this makes their present passive. Thinking too much about past deeds cannot be a reason for changes. Neither it creates something concrete nor makes your present productive. The only thing you can get from your past is an experience, which will make you aware and this awareness will guide you to make the right move, if the same incident happens again in your life.

Our positive thoughts will become our inspiration to perform better in our life. So, one should be always optimistic about life. Life becomes beautiful, if we live it beautifully.

In one of the scientific experiments, it is found that how our thoughts changes into faith and that faith becomes the cause of our present results. It is very famous and commonly known to all. Yes, you are right! We are talking about the medical experiment, in which 100 patients are given the best medicine as a remedy but it is said that no medicine can work to cure you. And another 100 patients got sugar-coated tablets as a medicine but it is pretended that they are getting the best medicine in the world and soon they are going to be cured. And as an astonishment, it is found that earlier patients with the best medicine got more sickness and other patients recovered from the sickness and became fit and fine.

This is the magic of our thoughts so, whenever you paint your dreams try to choose the best and amazing colours to make your life colourful and lively. This magical thinking will lead you towards the best life experiences. So, what are you waiting for? Start thinking bigger by doing every   day   better.

10. HAVE PATIENCE

Having patience in life is the most important thing. We wish, we put all our efforts and achieve our target and but sometimes we get an experience as things could be done better. This is the time of your real test in life. Life is all about ups and downs. Every night is followed by a bright sunny day which is a source of our happiness and liveliness. In the same way, time always does not remain same. It keeps changing. You need to handle this situation tactfully. This is the time you should have enough patience to move forward in life. If you get disturbed then you won't be able to take the right decision. Being calm and quiet will lead you to make a proper decision and plan. And this is the way you will come out of a problem. Be a warier. Warier does not afraid and never complaint but deals the situation with proper plan and continuous efforts and patience.

Here, one thing you need to understand that is having patience does not mean that be passive. You have to put efforts to be successful. For that, the first thing is having proper planning, keep ready Plan A and Plan B. If Plan A does not work then work on the Plan B, but before choosing it, give you 100% efforts to achieve Plan A. Second thing, deal the situation with patience. And the third thing, have faith upon your efforts. Right efforts with right strategies will always lead you to achieve your goal.

This is a time to play strategic war to achieve your aim so be smart, try to do things differently so that in a short time you can achieve many things.

CONCLUSION

Now, it's time to act. Habits you need to be a successful person are with you. Follow these things in your life to change your life more positively. These are the things that will help you when you apply them in your life. Only reading will just make you understand but following them will certainly create magic. Having faith is the next thing. These things will work definitely. Magic won't happen in a day, for that you have to make certain efforts and have patience until it happens. Life is a mysterious thing; hence, following certain principles and disciplines will lead you towards the happy journey of life.

To follow these habits, self-discipline is the best polity. No other person can change your life unless your craving for transformation. A person should always be motivated and this comes from self-discipline. Your self-will will keep you to keep yourself motivated. Always remember that you are the one who keeps observing yourself rather than any other person. Whatever thing you do, do it with discipline. Never think that this is just a small thing or how big it is. Things won't matter but the one thing that matters most is YOU. By following it you can achieve the things which you want. For that you have to start first with small things such as waking up at right time, get enough sleep, try to avoid excess use of technology, set time to be active social media, if it's necessary or unavoidable, complete the things which you star, set time limit to perform different tasks, follow your time, e.g. if you have to reach at a particular place then be on time. Time is the most precious thing in life. If you respect time then time will respect you. So, be the master of yourself and lead your life the way you want.

So, what are you waiting for? Start developing these habits from today onwards. Feel the happiness within you and observe the changes. Life is beautiful as it full of amazing and wonderful people like you. This is the new beginning my dear friends. In this journey of happiness, my best wishes are always with you. Stay happy and stay blessed.

***

ABOUT THE AUTHOR

This book is written by Pramod Dhumale. By profession, he is an Assistant Professor. He has been working as a teacher for the last 11 years. He is a well-known teacher, motivational speaker, blogger, content writer, translator and newspaper columnist. He has published several research papers in national and international research journals. And above all, he always strives for the welfare for the human beings.